Lifestyle Matters

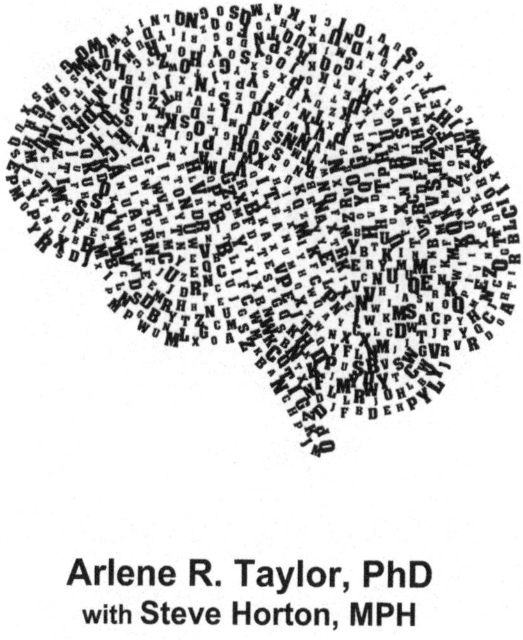

Arlene R. Taylor, PhD
with Steve Horton, MPH

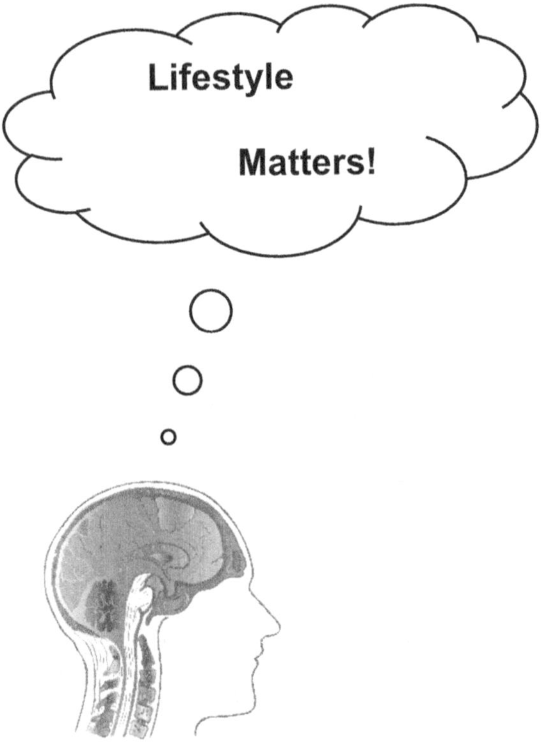
Lifestyle
Matters!

Lifestyle Matters

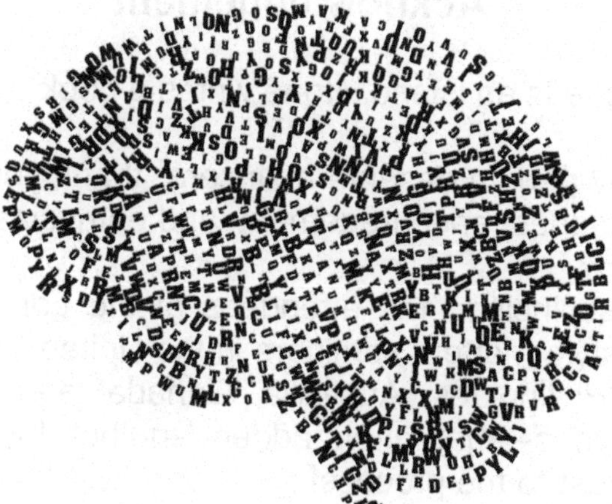

Arlene R. Taylor, PhD
with Steve Horton, MPH

Success Resources International
Napa, CA, USA

Dedication

This book is dedicated to all those who want to understand how much lifestyle really matters, especially for those who aim to stay healthier and younger for longer.

Acknowledgement

No one is an island. None writes a book alone.

Many people deserve a sincere "thank you" for their ideas, encouragement, and enthusiasm.

These include the attendees at the Longevity Lifestyle Matters seminars in the United States, the Philippines, Australia, Canada, and other locations—that often added another layer of interest to the process!

Address requests for information to:
Arlene R. Taylor, PhD
310 Crawford Way, P.O. Box #10187
American Canyon, CA 94503-1113 USA

ISBN: 978-1-957390-99-4

Cover picture by openclipart.com Used by permission

Appendix: 7 Case Studies collected and written by Joeveney Macabeo, PhD
Lydia Bautista, DNP, DipACLM, counselor for case studies #1-6; Cherie Lou Fernandez, MD, counselor for case study #7. Used by permission. Pseudonyms are used to protect privacy.

Book production & cover by David Eastman
Printed in the United States of America

Publisher's Reminder

Lifestyle Matters is provided for general educational and informational purposes only and does not present an in-depth treatment of specific research findings or topics. The information is not intended to take the place of professional counseling, medical or psychological care, recovery therapy, or personalized recommendations from healthcare professionals. Since every brain is different, there are no guarantees of individual results.

Be sure to consult your physician or other healthcare professionals before you make lifestyle changes or implement new exercise strategies. The publisher, authors, contributors, reviewers, editors, certified facilitators, or volunteers expressly disclaim all responsibility and any liability whatsoever (direct or indirect) for outcomes or adverse effects (actual or perceived), from use, misuse, or inappropriate application of concepts presented herein.

Someone was heard to say that "No book ever written is completely without mistakes." If you find typos, please know that they do serve a purpose. Making mistakes is part and parcel of being human—and some brains really enjoy hunting for mistakes.

Table of Contents

If you keep on doing what you are doing, you will keep on getting what you are getting.

—George E. Guthrie, MD, MPH

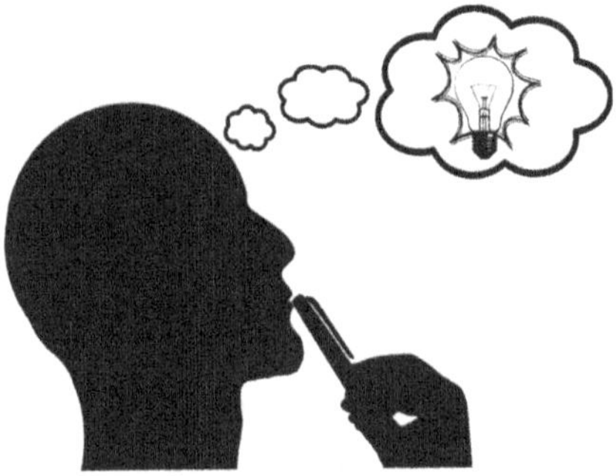

As soon as you start to change your lifestyle for the better, you will begin to repair yesterday's damage.

—Gary W. Small, MD

Introduction

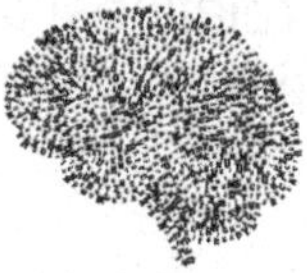

Lifestyle begins in the brain. Many factors impact how human beings choose their lifestyle. Current wisdom is that many lifestyle choices have proven unhelpful in assisting individuals to stay healthier and younger for longer.

Unfortunately, the lifestyle choices that were made shortened lifespans in some cases.

Estimates are that this generation may be the first to live shorter lives than their parents—largely attributed to lifestyle choices.

Fortunately, studies are showing that there are ways to stay healthier and younger for longer. While altering habits and beliefs may be a challenge, it is doable. Your brain's glymphatic immune system, hand-in-glove and your body's general immune system, work to keep you well and if you get sick, to help you heal.

Information is provided as little bites. Read a few at a time and ask yourself, "Given this information, is there something I am able to turn into knowledge and practically apply in my life to help me stay heathier and younger for longer?" If yes, make the necessary adjustments.

Chapters 15 and 16 are included for those who desire more information on Alzheimer's prevention and on the close relationship between genetics and epigenetics, which includes lifestyle.

The Appendix contains seven case studies of real people who altered their lifestyle and the results they experienced.

Bottom line?

Lifestyle matters!

—Arlene & Steve

*****

This is why Lifestyle Matters:

70% of how long and how well you live is in your hands.

—Michael A. Roisen, MD & Mehmet C. Oz, MD

1 - Mindset

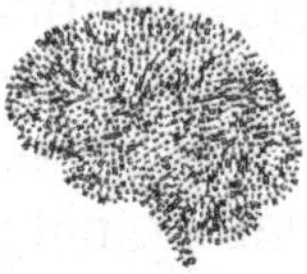

Doc Lew Childre Jr., and Howard Martin of the *HeartMath Institute*, wrote that your habitual attitudes form neural circuits (or pathways) in the brain. If you choose to maintain a specific attitude, the brain can literally rewire itself to facilitate that attitude.

Everything begins in your brain! The choices you make automatically or by conscious choice are all influenced by your mindset. Kendra Cherry, MSEd, defined mindset as a set of beliefs that affect how you see yourself and the world.

In her book, *Mindset,* Carol S. Dweck, PhD, pointed out that two different mindsets exist. A fixed mindset believes that one's abilities are fixed traits and therefore cannot be changed. A fixed mindset seldom solves anything. It can even create more problems if it triggers a stress response such as Fight-Flight

A *growth* mindset on the other hand says: "My brain can learn and improve. It's my job to make it happen." A growth mindset believes that your talents and abilities can be identified, developed, and honed over time through your efforts and persistence.

Dr. Dweck and colleagues found that children behaved very differently depending on the type of praise they received. Praising a child's talents or labeling them as "smart," promoted a fixed mindset. It sent a message that the child either had an ability or did not and there was nothing they could do to change that. Process praise, on the other hand, emphasized the effort a child put in to accomplish a task, which implied their success was partly due to their own effort and the strategy they used, both of which they could control and improve over time.

A positive mindset plus consistent practical application of information that you have turned into knowledge can motivate you to apply it in a way that works for you, and that you will maintain for the rest of your life.

Only one idea can occupy your brain's working memory at a time. Negative thoughts trigger the recall of negative memories. Positive thoughts trigger the recall of positive memories and encourage you to stay positive and persevere.

Life experiences can influence the type of mindset you develop. So can the people you spend the most time with. Estimates are that 50% of the problems human beings experience are of their own making—based on the way they think. That's *mindset*. If you have an enemy outpost of negativity inside your brain, dump it! Unmanaged negative thinking creates a type of stress that is said to be the precursor of all life-threatening illnesses. A negative mindset adversely impacts all your relationships and your success potential. It also cripples a long, joyful, healthy, and productive life. Learn to recognize negative thoughts quickly and replace them with positive *can-do* thoughts.

Mindset alters your neurochemistry which, in turn, impacts your immune systems. Although mindset happens internally, what occurs outside your brain and body tends to mirror what is happening on the inside.

Your mindset has a way of aligning with either the negative *or* the positive. Those who are truly successful are known for being able to move from mistake to mistake with no loss of enthusiasm. They learn from their mistakes, as well as from the mistakes of others. You won't live long enough to make every mistake on your own.

Affirmations are positive, present-tense, words and phrases designed to impact both the conscious and subconscious minds. In turn, affirmations impact your mindset, self-talk, habits, and exhibited behaviors. Done correctly nothing else is as effective.

Jean Marie Stine put it this way: "Affirmation is the mind's programming language."

You are the only person who can flip the switch from a *fixed* to a *growth* mindset. Sometimes just doing that can make all the difference in the world—even impacting your lifespan. If you choose a growth mindset, your rate of making mistakes may decrease even as your rate of success increases.

As soon as you wake up in the morning, give thanks for something. Throughout the day, be grateful for every positive thing that happens, however small. Do a random act of kindness every day.

Maddy Malhotra wrote: "Either you control your thoughts or outside forces will; and be warned that the outside forces usually consist of fears, worries, and doubts."

Henry Ford, said: "Whether you think you can or whether you think you can't, you're right."

*****

Your self-talk is the channel of behavior change. —**Gino Norris**

2 - Self-talk

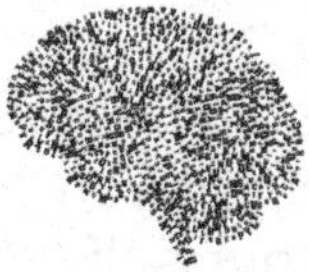

The term self-talk was first used in 1737 to describe the way human beings tend to communicate with themselves. It is label for what you tell yourself internally, silently, or aloud. It follows your mindset.

John Lembo has pointed out that each waking moment human beings talk to themselves about the things they experience in life. Their self-talk, the thoughts they communicate to themselves, controls the way they feel and act. Skeptical? Close your eyes for a few moments and listen to what you hear. Your thoughts.

Tell your brain only what you want to have happen as if it is already happening. Make your self-talk positive and present tense, as the brain tends to get in gear based on what is happening in the present moment. If you tell your brain, "Tomorrow I am going to …" the brain registers future tense and thinks *Tomorrow is then. This is now. When 'then' arrives, I'll help you.*

Positive self-talk helps you achieve your goals, increase your energy, attain better health, and potentially a longer lifespan. Negative self-talk drains energy and can trigger anxiety, illness, hopelessness, and undesirable behaviors.

Your mindset, beliefs, and what people say to you or what you heard them say about you all have a huge impact on your life. Your self-talk creates your reality, influencing your thoughts and feelings, and triggering your behaviors

Estimates are that the average person, growing up in a moderately functional family, heard 10 negative words for every positive word. In a less functional family, the ratio may be more like 30-40 negatives to every positive.

It will take some practice to over-ride those old *messages* playing inside your head. Metaphorically, learn to reach up and turn down the volume when you "hear" or "think" about negative words from your past.

Research by Ethan Kross, PhD, found that using distanced self-talk—referring to oneself in the 3rd person—can enhance emotional control and problem-solving abilities. This approach helps create psychological distance, which can improve mood and focus, especially in high-pressure situations. Use your given *name* (so the brain knows who is talking) followed by the words *you are* and what you want your brain to do—in present-tense words.

For example: "Joe, you are drinking a glass of water before eating." "Jill, you are giving your brain positive words and instructions."

The brain's and body's *energy* are closely linked with self-talk, and the internal mental pictures your words create. Positive self-talk patterns can strengthen your brain's and body's immune systems and boost energy levels. Negative self-talk patterns can do the opposite. Anger and anxiety are energy eaters.

Your brain can only do what it thinks it can do, and it's your job to tell it what it can do. Your conscious mind listens to and believes what you say *to* and *about* yourself. Your subconscious mind doesn't use language per se, but it follows the pictures your self-talk creates. It believes that *if* you say it and *if* you picture it, you must want it.

Shad Helmstetter reported that the brain simply believes what you tell most about yourself. Therefore, the conscious mind creates a mental picture in working memory of what it thinks you want—for the subconscious mind to follow.

Jon Gordon, MA, author of *The Energy Bus,* has advised: "Speak positively first thing in the morning, and your energy will increase."

Avoid using words like *can't* and *don't* and *won't*, as they do not tell your brain what to do. Give your brain *positive* instructions to achieve *positive* outcomes. It's the difference between saying, "Don't touch the stove" (which creates a picture of touching the stove) versus "Keep your hands away from the stove" (which creates a picture of the behavior you want exhibited).

David Taylor-Klaus has been quoted as saying, "Words matter, and the words that matter most are the ones you say to yourself."

Positive self-talk is less stressful and more effective. It reduces anxiety and requires less electrical activity.

Stop telling yourself what you do not want to have happen and talk only about what you do want to have happen—as if it's already a done deal and is in the bag.

*****

What really matters for success, character, happiness, and life-long achievements is a definite set of emotional skills—your EQ—not just purely cognitive abilities that are measured by conventional IQ tests.

—Daniel J. Goleman, PhD

3 - IQ versus EQ

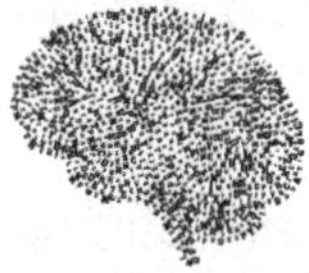

Living successfully appears to be *a* combination of IQ (intelligence quotient) and EQ (Emotional Intelligence). IQ represents your potential academic achievement. You inherit IQ from your biological parents, whether you lived with them or not. EQ is not inherited. It represents how you manage your emotions, feelings, relationships, self-awareness, and leadership activities. EQ is developed by you and your brain together.

According to David Caruso, it is critically important to understand that EQ is not the opposite of IQ. It is not the triumph of heart over head—it is the unique intersection of both.

Mean IQ scores in the US have fallen from 100 to 98 in the last few years. Some have suggested this relates to the increased use of technology. It has been said that 98 is 62 points lower than Einstein's estimated IQ of 160.

In his book *Emotional Intelligence*, Daniel J. Goleman, PhD, wrote that one's IQ potential, at best, contributes only about 20% to the factors that help determine a person's overall success. EQ, on the other hand, can be much more powerful, likely contributing 80% or more to one's success in life. This may help to explain the reason some individuals with reportedly high IQ's realize little success in life—their EQ is not nearly as high as their IQ.

Triggered by internal or external stimuli, emotions connect the conscious mind with the subconscious mind, offering both information and energy. In the grip of a strong emotion, the brain (seeking congruity) tends to recall past events that involved a similar emotion, intensifying the present emotion.

High EQ can help you identify core emotions quickly, recognize the information they provide, and manage them effectively. High EQ also helps you manage the feelings created by your brain's interpretation of what the emotions are trying to convey. You are not responsible for every emotion that arises. You are responsible for the feelings you choose to hang onto since your brain creates them. If you don't like the way you *feel*, change the way you *think*—because feelings always follow emotions and thoughts.

Teams led by consistently demonstrate 20% higher productivity and 67% better collaboration (compared with teams led by low EQ leaders). High EQ leaders can present information and strategies in a non-threatening manner, allowing for input from various opinion segments. They can look ahead and estimate if today's proposed solution(s) will still be relevant a few years down the line or may require a different solution.

High EQ helps you evaluate a situation as quickly and accurately as possible and determine what action (if any) is needed. It helps you estimate how much a given event will really matter in 12 months. If probability is high, start problem-solving. If low, let it go.

When asked for your opinion, high EQ allows you to share as honestly and graciously as possible, while remaining relatively indifferent as to whether your opinion is accepted. This helps you avoid badgering others to embrace your perspective.

Uterine scans have observed at least four emotions—joy, anger, fear, and sadness—on fetal faces during gestation. There are scores of descriptors for these emotions. All core emotions are innately positive, although exhibited behaviors are often negative.

PET scans showed that the emotion of joy lights up the brain's left hemisphere. The three "protective" emotions of anger, fear, and sadness light up the right hemisphere. Joy indicates that life is basically going well. Anger alerts you that your boundaries have been breached. Fear warns that you may be in danger (unless it is an imaginary fear). Sadness confirms you have suffered a loss and helps you recover and feel better again.

JOT behaviors represent low EQ. Estimates are that they may be responsible for at least 70% of all misunderstandings and conflicts. JOT behaviors are: Jumping to conclusions, Overreacting, and Taking things personally.

Use AAA replacement behaviors to minimize JOT behaviors. AAA stands for: Ask questions to clarify the situation; Act calmly as you assess the situation to determine if there is anything you need to do; Avoid taking things personally by altering your perception, as the event or situation may have nothing to do with you.

Unfortunately, hospitals, institutions, and prisons are filled with individuals who did not—or were unable to handle their emotions and feelings effectively and appropriately.

*****

Those who think they have no time for bodily exercise will sooner or later have to find time for illness. —Edward Stanley

4 - Physical Exercise

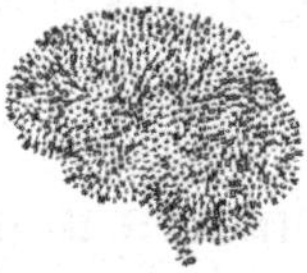

Basic physical exercise is vitally important for the health of the human brain and body. It strengthens the heart, bolsters the immune systems, boosts energy, relieves stress, enhances cognition, and improves sleep.

The value of exercise has less to do with building muscles or burning calories and more to do with getting the heart to pump faster and more efficiently, thereby increasing blood flow to nourish and cleanse the brain and body organs.

The exercise of large muscle groups facilitates the return of blood to the heart through the veins and the return of lymph fluid through the lymph vessels.

Blood circulates through the body about once a minute—at sometimes two or three times a minute depending on your heart rate and activity. Each day, every cell in the blood travels a distance nearly half-way around Planet Earth at its equator!

When operating correctly, the circulatory system is a very effective two-way distribution system. It delivers oxygen, glucose, and other essential !micronutrients to each cell. In turn, it picks up carbon dioxide, carrying it (and other waste products) away. Without exercise these essential tasks may not be accomplished effectively.

The World Health Organization estimates that 35% of the world's billions of people are not getting enough physical exercise. Females are estimated to get even less exercise than males,

Studies of senior citizens who walk regularly (as compared to sedentary elderly people) showed improvement in memory skills, learning ability, concentration, and abstract reasoning.

According to Candace B. Pert, PhD, 20 minutes of mild aerobic exercise at the beginning of the day turns on fat-burning neuropeptides, the effects of which can last for hours. This can be critical in managing diseases such as obesity and diabetes. The book *Brain Rules* explains that upping your daily exercise to a 20-minute walk could cut stroke risk by 57%.

Minimize *sitting* and maximize *moving*. If you are doing largely sedentary work, do some standing at a raised desk, if possible. Move around for a couple of minutes every half hour, setting a timer if need be. Aim to exercise for 30 minutes each day, in sections of 10 or 15 minutes if that works better for your schedule.

Include stretching, aerobics, endurance, balance, and flexibility exercises.

Many say they "hate" exercising. That is an unhelpful mindset. Studies have shown that when you "hate" something, doing it anyway does not provide the benefits that can be accrued if you are on board with it. Identify what you already do: vacuuming, washing the car, cutting the grass, biking, walking, swimming, doing the laundry, cleaning house, and so on.

There are only two requirements when it comes to exercise according to Jennie Brand-Miller. One is that you do it; the other is that you continue to do it.

Willpower can be defined as the energetic determination to carry out your chosen plans and decisions. Not designed to stop bad habits, especially those that light up the Brain Reward System, willpower is designed to help you create a new behavior. Picture in your mind what you plan to do for exercise, then use willpower to help you do it.

Use it and move it or *lose* it—but choose your physical activities and exercise routines with care. The advice of Hippocrates still stands: *Do no harm.* For example, after decades of being touted as beneficial, jogging (as compared with brisk walking or running) is getting very mixed reviews for the average person. Over time, jogging can damage joints, stretch ligaments, and may even compound cellulite.

Physical exercise is an anti-aging strategy. Variety is key to keeping your brain interested and motivated, so select activities and exercises you enjoy. Be creative. Even small changes can contribute to enhanced health and longevity. Nearly everyone can find some way to obtain their needed physical activity and exercise.

Concentrate on what you can do. Stop fretting about what you no longer can do, using that as an excuse for laziness.

Research suggests that 30 minutes of physical activity and exercise plus 30 minutes of challenging mental activity and activity each day is a desirable goal. Imagine what 30 + 30 could do for you!

*****

Exercise does seem to reduce the risk of developing Alzheimer's disease, as well as other forms of dementia or other causes of cognitive decline.

—Neuropsychiatrist Dylan Wint, MD

5 - Brain Exercise

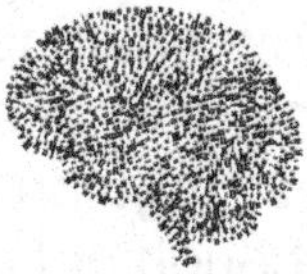

According to Richard Restak, MD, physical exercise is the single most powerful tool you have to optimize your brain function. It can improve creativity, concentration, problem-solving, and help delay the onset of any memory loss. It prepares your neurons to connect with each other, while mental stimulation allows your brain to capitalize on that readiness.

Brain exercises involve challenging the neurons (thinking cells) in your brain. The dendrites are covered with tiny hairs that receive and pull information into the cell. Information leaves a neuron through the axon. Neurotransmitters transfer the information across the synapse (space) between neurons, as they do not touch each other. Hopefully, the information is picked up by a neuron on the other side of the synapse. If not stimulated on a regular basis, neurons, along with their axons and dendrites, can atrophy or shrink. This widens the synapse, making the transfer of information from one neuron to another more difficult or even impossible. If information does not get transferred to other neurons, symptoms of dementia can develop.

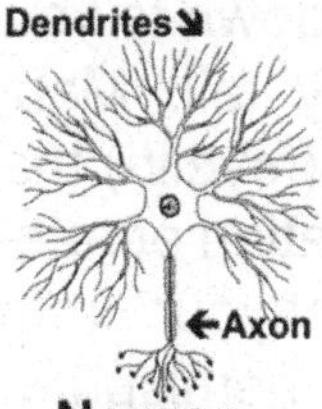

Neuron

Imagine a leafless tree in winter. That's what a neuron can look like when it has not regularly received challenging stimulation. Now imagine a beautiful maple tree in full leaf. That's what a neuron can look like when it has regularly received challenging stimulation. Although not a muscle, the brain responds much like muscle tissue. Use it or lose it.

Studies have shown that dendrites can alter their shape in 30 seconds. Neurons can grow a new dendrite in 30 minutes—depending on the amount of stimulation they receive.

Some axons reach from your brain down to your toes—a long way if you are very tall! Many axons are wrapped with insulation (myelin) that helps speed transmission of information at rates up to 600 mph (985 km/h) in parts of your brain. This is especially true in the right hemisphere where more white matter exists. (The left hemisphere contains more gray matter.)

Studies by Veterans showed that those who were apathetic (i.e., showed indifference) were up to seven times more likely to develop dementia. Estimates are that about 15% of individuals age 65 and older who are diagnosed with pre-dementia will go on to evidence full-blown dementia. Some studies have shown that when brains with pre-dementia are helped to challenge their brains using mental games, reading, listening to audio books, singing, and whistling, combined with physical activity on a daily basis, the development of symptoms could be slowed and sometimes even reversed if caught early.

Brain stimulation is essential for a healthy brain and critical for the aging brain. Do something every day to keep your brain interested! Avoid zoning out in front of the TV, just passively processing what another brain created. Maximize active mental picturing by engaging in stimulating and challenging mental activities for at least 30 minutes a day to keep your brain active and your synapses narrow.

Play mental games and word games. There are some excellent word quizzes on TV that can challenge the brain. Assemble puzzles.

Read aloud for at least 10-15 minutes a day to promote brain-function activity.

Listen to audio books. Hone your creativity in every way possible!

Travel (locally, nationally, internationally) if you can. Expose your brain to new sights, sounds, smells, tastes, people, and environments.

Develop a challenging and rewarding hobby. Volunteer in a genre that interests you.

Learn to use a computer and do internet searches.

Listen to positive cheerful music. Music is one of the few activities that stimulates, activates, and engages the entire brain.

Anita Collins, PhD, an award-winning educator, researcher, and writer, is internationally recognized for her unique work in translating the scientific research of neuroscientists and psychologists to the everyday parent, teacher, and student. She has explained that when you listen to music, multiple areas of the brain become engaged and active. When you play a musical instrument, however, it becomes more like a full-on brain-body workout with fireworks!

Children who take music lessons before age seven have larger corpus callosum bridges between the hemispheres. The research is solid. If you don't play a musical instrument, start learning one now. The benefits can lead to a healthier retirement and even a longer lifespan.

*****

Sleep is independently linked with longevity.
—Institute of Natural Resources

6 - Sleep & Lifespan

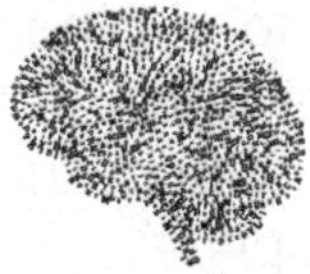

Sleep deprivation is pandemic on Planet Earth. Estimates are that 80% of the world's population needs an alarm clock to wake up. More than 80 million Americans are sleep deprived—their brains are not getting the optimum sleep needed to accomplish required functions. Contributing factors may relate to the invention of electric lights and the proliferation of electronic equipment—which can cause a mismatch between biology and technology.

Alex Dimitriu, MD, has pointed out that sleep has a powerful role to play in brain health. Sleep is essential for the body to rest but is even more important for the brain to declutter. At night, the brain processes the events of the day. It transfers memories into long-term storage and makes room for new learning on the next day.

Your brain does not *rest* while you sleep, since hundreds of biological processes continue. Some brain areas are more active and work harder while you are asleep than when you are awake. This is due to a myriad of critical housekeeping chores that typically require at least 7-8 hours for the brain to accomplish—for an estimated majority of adults.

Imagine hiring a cleaning service where the workers routinely leave an hour or two before their shift is over. As they continue to cut their work time short, it doesn't take long for "unfinished tasks" to accumulate. Soon the workers are too far behind to catch up!

In his book *Why We Sleep,* Matthew Walker wrote that sleep is not an optional lifestyle luxury. It is a non-negotiable biological necessity. For every period of exhaustion, a corresponding period of depression can derail optimum brain function.

During sleep, human growth hormones are produced. Electricity is generated for thinking and energy production. Hormones, neurotransmitters, enzymes, and other chemicals are replenished. Food for the neurons (neurotrophins) is made, cells are repaired, metabolic waste is excreted, and the immune systems are strengthened.

During sleep, the brain can experiment without inhibition, often coming up with never-before-imagined ideas. An optimum amount of sleep lowers one's risk for dementia, depression, psychosis, and stroke. Lack of sleep can drain one's energy, interfere with effective decision-making and problem-solving, increase mistakes, raise a risk for accidents, trigger weight gain, increase irritability, and accelerate aging.

Sleep is essential for all healthy memory functions. Insufficient sleep will interfere with all types of memory functions. This includes declarative memory, implicit non-declarative memory, and creative or intelligent memory.

When awake and exposed to new information, the brain shoves what it learns into short-term memory banks. During sleep, the brain consolidates the information. Think of the hippocampus (the brain's search engine) as rewinding and replaying what happened during the day for the cerebrum to review. Information is either discarded or moved into long-term storage.

When you consciously want to retrieve a memory, the hippocampus searches for and (hopefully) locates the information—if it was moved into long-term memory, that is.

An hour before bedtime, turn off all blue-light-emitting diodes or LEDs (unless you have been wearing special glasses that block the blue light from entering your eyes). Blue light suppresses melatonin production and increases alertness—exactly what you do *not* want when you *do* want to sleep.

Melatonin is a hormone that impacts sleep and regulates biological rhythms. Light from any source slows the release of melatonin from the pineal gland. Sleep in as dark a room as possible. Consider wearing eye coverings. Any light, however brief, can slow or even shut down melatonin production.

Remove all electronic products from the bedroom such as televisions and computers. The electrical energy they produce can disturb the brain as it is trying to sleep. If you need an alarm, consider using a small wind-up or battery clock that does not exhibit a light.

Sleep has been called the "golden chain" that ties your health and body together. Give your brain and body the *optimum* amount of sleep they need.

The loss of just one hour of sleep per night on a regular basis can—and some researchers say will—shorten your lifespan.

*****

Water deprivation kills faster than the lack of any other nutrient.

—Linda Boeckner & Kay McKinzie

7 – Hydration & Energy

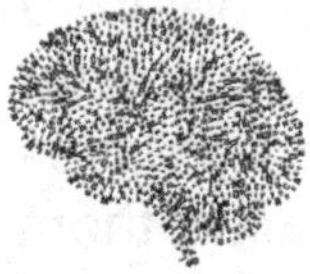

Estimates are that most people over age 50 drink less than 1 quart (32 oz) or 1 liter of water per day. The average adult loses more than 80 oz of water daily through sweating, breathing, and waste elimination, which puts the individual 48 ounces in deficit compared to the amount of water taken in. Some children and adults drink mostly sodas (regular or diet), fruit juices, sugary drinks, tea, coffee, or cola.

Body organs will sacrifice their need for water in favor of the brain, even dehydrating urine and sending the liquid up to the brain (making it a "pee" brain). Unless medically contraindicated, drink enough pure water for one or two pale urines daily.

Marjie Gilliam has said that water is your body's most important nutrient. It is involved in every brain-body function, and accounts for 70-75% of your total body weight. Water helps you maintain body temperature, metabolize body fat, digest your food, lubricate and cushion internal organs, transport nutrients, and flush toxins from your body.

Make pure water your "beverage of choice," as it is absorbed quickly and needs no digestion. Drink a glass of water 15-30 minutes before a meal to help ensure you are eating from hunger rather than from thirst. The water also increases the fluidity of digestive juices and helps them handle the food you eat more efficiently.

Corinne Allen, PhD, founder of the Advanced Learning & Development Institute, has explained that brain cells require twice the energy that other cells in the body need. Water provides this energy more effectively than any other substance. Individuals with brain challenges such as autism spectrum, ADD, ADHD, head injuries, anxiety attacks, and depression, often drink little or no water. The lack of water exacerbates brain dysfunction.

Dehydration shrinks brain cells. If dehydration continues, brain tissue can pull away from the skull. This is linked with an increased risk for developing dementia.

1% dehydration results in a 5% decrease in mental acuity. This cognitive reduction may lead to difficulties making change while shopping, navigating around town, or deciding between two options. 2% dehydration can result in memory loss and difficulty with mathematical calculations.

Dehydration kills faster than the lack of any other nutrient. You can live at least 10 times longer without food than without water. Like estimates of the composition of Planet Earth, body and brain average about one fourth solid matter and three-fourths water, with brain neurons containing higher percentages. Even bones are about 20% water! Dehydration is an alteration in this ratio toward solid matter.

Dehydration impacts all brain-body systems, but it is especially lethal to brain function, slowing it down and interfering with vital thinking processes. Many adults over 60 are believed to be chronically dehydrated.

Normally, there is more water inside a cell than outside. Dehydration reverses that ratio. Water generates electrical energy for all brain functions. The movement of water in and out of the cells functions much like a hydroelectric plant. The energy created is stored as adenosine triphosphate (ATP), the cell's main energy source. Brain cells are said to need three times the water that is required by muscle tissue. Water provides this energy more effectively than any other substance. When water levels fall, energy production also falls.

Dehydration can cause brain tissue to shrink and pull away from the skull; a condition now linked with dementia. It is also associated with lymph fluid problems, low blood volume, increased risk of clotting, headaches, irritability, inflammation, kidney failure, heat cramps, heatstroke, depression, and seizures due to electrolyte loss. Dehydration produces free radicals that wrinkle the skin, as well as wrinkling internal body organs.

Many children grow up being given food when they are fussy instead of first being offered water to see if they are thirsty—or physiologically hungry. Consequently, many never learn to differentiate between genuine physiological hunger and thirst. In addition, because thirst sensation tends to fall with age, it is not a reliable sign of dehydration.

Several studies suggest that drinking hydrogen water may reduce inflammation, decrease oxidative stress, improve athletic performance, and provide antioxidant properties, et cetera.

*****

Accidents will still happen no matter how many safeguards are put into place. However, this doesn't mean that a majority cannot be prevented.

—Fromthegreennotebook.com

8 – Brain-Body Safety

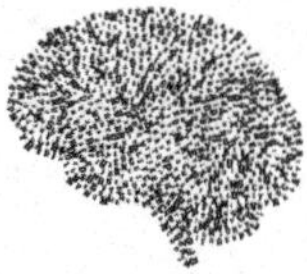

Did you know that Brain Safety Awareness Day is celebrated in the United States on March 4th?

You only have one brain. No replacement is available. It's prevention all the way. You only have one body, too. While a few body-organ replacements exist, they are often less efficient than the originals. Safety is important for both brain and body since, as Thomas Edison put it, the chief function of your body is to carry your brain around. A functional brain in a diseased or damaged body can often accomplish a great deal. A damaged or diseased brain in an otherwise functional body? Not so much.

Typically, brain neurons (thinking cells) do not replace themselves by dividing and multiplying as do most other body cells. Therefore, many of your brain's neurons may be the same ones you had at birth. Safety includes paying attention to the researched strategies related to health and longevity of these vital neurons in both your brain and body.

Broken bones, traumatic brain injuries, sexually transmitted diseases, and many addictive behaviors can cut short a life that might have lived and thrived successfully for another decade or more. Be proactive about safety. *Knowing* is one thing. *Implementing* what you know is another. While genuine accidents do occur, prevention, which isn't rocket science, can be very helpful. Estimates are that over half of all accidents were avoidable.

Protect your head. Avoid concussions and skull fractures by avoiding unsafe activities and refusing to take dares. Some dare devils may be willing to risk life and limb, but you don't need to.

Avoid distracted walking and driving. Many get into accidents during distractions.

As far as possible, avoid exposure to radiation, toxins, poisons, any substances known to be harmful to brain or body, and transmissible infectious diseases. Avoid substances that may damage the brain's neuronal control centers.

Protect your mind. Avoid exposing it to negative pictures, images, or ideas that might return to disturb sleep, trigger nightmares, or any undesirable behavior that might result in injury—like falling out of bed or falling down the stairs.

Protect your lungs. Inhale fresh air, minimize exposure to pollutants such as tobacco smoke, vehicle exhaust, and fire smoke. Wear a mask if air quality is poor.

Protect your ears when around loud sounds.

Protect your eyes when involved in activities that could trigger flying debris.

Protect your digestive system from low-quality foods and beverages—from *anything* that could diminish its effectiveness.

Wear a seat belt every time you are in any type of motor vehicle. Never drive while under the influence of alcohol or drugs.

Fall-proof your home. Remove throw rugs and other tripping hazards. Use a sturdy stepstool when reaching for high objects. Be careful with ladders—stay off them and off the roof. (Leave that to the experts!)

The first time you do something, your brain lays out the outline of new software in case you want to do it again. The good news is that this makes repeating that behavior easier. The bad news is that the brain can end up developing some bad habits because you "did something once."

Wear a helmet or appropriate headgear any time you are doing any activity where there is the possibility of falling and hitting your head like horseback riding, surfing, skiing, skating, or riding in all-terrain vehicles.

Choose a sports program that enforces rules for safety and avoids drills and plays that increase the risk for head impact.

A smart man only believes half of what he hears. A wise man knows which half ... Safety is something that happens between your ears, and not something you hold in your hands.

—Jeff Cooper

The NFL acknowledges that repetitive trauma to the head in football ... can cause a permanent, disabling injury to the brain. —Bob Fitzsimmons

An ounce of prevention is worth a pound of cure.

—Benjamin Franklin

Making safe, wise choices about brain-body safety means that you are planning for a healthier future. What you do today determines where you will be tomorrow.

*****

Healthy exposure to sunlight can boost the production of serotonin, the happy hormone that also makes you feel calmer and more focused and optimistic. The sun always shines above the clouds.

—Paul F. Davis

9 - Sunlight 101

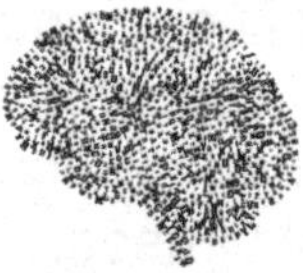

Much of life could not exist on Planet Earth without sunlight. When and how much exposure is obtained, however, can be a critical factor in terms of one's health. Estimates are that one in five Americans will develop skin cancer during their lifetime. Research emphasizes the importance of using sunscreen daily, wearing protective clothing, and seeking shade during peak sunshine hours to prevent sun damage. Wear a hat when at the beach and use sunglasses in bright sunlight to lower your risk of developing macular degeneration.

According to Mandeep Kaur, MD, skin cancer appears to be the most rapidly growing cause of cancer deaths in the US. Prevention of both melanoma and non-melanoma skin cancer needs to begin in childhood. Reduction in childhood sunlight exposure and tanning will hopefully stem the rise of skin cancer.

Exposing one's arms to natural light for an estimated 10-15 minutes a day can provide the needed benefits for some skin types. Dark skin, however, may need quite a bit more exposure to natural light than does light skin. *Excessive* exposure is defined as inappropriate amounts of exposure to ultraviolet radiation (UVR) for an individual's skin type and color. Excessive and unprotected exposure to sunlight can contribute to premature aging, skin wrinkling, and cataracts. It is also linked with conditions aggravated by immunosuppression, which allows the reactivation of some latent viruses.

Entrainment is a label for the process of keeping your brain's circadian rhythm clock in sync with the sun. In the morning as sunlight enters the eyes, light sensitive cells in the retina send electrical signals to the suprachiasmatic nucleus (SCN) in the brain's hypothalamus, which wakes up body organs and notifies the pineal gland to stop secreting the hormone melatonin.

If light cannot get to the retina, the cycle of the circadian rhythm clock begins to lengthen beyond approximately 24 hours. "Non-24-hour sleep-wake disorder" is rare in brains with normal visual functions. However, it is common in brains with total blindness, because the SCN does not receive the light that triggers entrainment.

At sundown, the SCN tells the pineal gland to release melatonin, the hormone that helps to regulate one's sleep-wake cycle, promoting a sense of being sleepy. Exposing the brain to artificial light after sundown can interrupt the release of melatonin.

Different from melatonin, melanin is a pigment responsible for the color of your skin, hair, and eyes. Melanin can provide some protection against UV radiation. Beyond the known effects related to Vitamin D production and calcium utilization, sunlight turns on internal chemical reactions and stimulates enzymes to work more effectively.

Major Depressive Disorder with Seasonal Pattern (formerly Seasonal Affective Disorder or SAD) is linked with insufficient exposure to ambient sunlight. It is more common in areas of the world farther from the equator due to greater seasonal variations in daylight hours. Brain plasticity and depression, regulated in part by Brain-Derived Neurotrophic Factor (BDNF), are also linked with the amount of ambient sunlight.

Some teenagers experience a sleep-phase delay. Their melatonin levels naturally rise later at night (compared with many other children and adults). These adolescents feel alert later in evening and may find it difficult to fall asleep before eleven o'clock or even midnight. Sleep deprivation, compounded by early school start-times, can negatively impact their life in general and *learning* in particular. Tips include turning off electronics an hour before bedtime (or wearing special glasses to block LED light), keeping lights dim as bedtime approaches, and obtaining exposure to bright light as soon as possible in the morning.

Jet lag results from the disruption of the circadian rhythm clock as the brain passes through different time zones, putting it in conflict with normal sleep patterns. The severity of jet lag often increases with the number of time zones crossed. Jet lag is generally more pronounced when traveling eastward. On average, it takes the brain about one day to adjust for each time zone crossed. If possible, start using the time at your destination a couple of days before hopping on the plane.

According to the Skin Cancer Foundation high-pressure sunlamps used in tanning salons generate UVA doses up to 12 times more than the sun. Clients are 2.5 times more likely to develop squamous cell carcinomas and 1.5 times more likely to develop basal cell carcinomas. Exposure to tanning beds in one's youth can increase the risk of developing melanoma by 75%.

*****

The food you eat can either be the safest and most powerful form of medicine, or the slowest form of poison.

—Ann Wigmore

8 – Brain-Body Safety

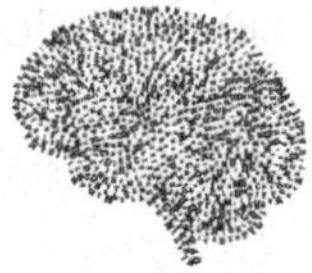

Did you know that Brain Safety Awareness Day is celebrated in the United States on March 4th?

You only have one brain. No replacement is available. It's prevention all the way. You only have one body, too. While a few body-organ replacements exist, they are often less efficient than the originals. Safety is important for both brain and body since, as Thomas Edison put it, the chief function of your body is to carry your brain around. A functional brain in a diseased or damaged body can often accomplish a great deal. A damaged or diseased brain in an otherwise functional body? Not so much.

Typically, brain neurons (thinking cells) do not replace themselves by dividing and multiplying as do most other body cells. Therefore, many of your brain's neurons may be the same ones you had at birth. Safety includes paying attention to the researched strategies related to health and longevity of these vital neurons in both your brain and body.

Broken bones, traumatic brain injuries, sexually transmitted diseases, and many addictive behaviors can cut short a life that might have lived and thrived successfully for another decade or more. Be proactive about safety. *Knowing* is one thing. *Implementing* what you know is another. While genuine accidents do occur, prevention, which isn't rocket science, can be very helpful. Estimates are that over half of all accidents were avoidable.

Protect your head. That is where your brain lives! Avoid concussions and skull fractures by avoiding unsafe activities and refusing to take a dare. Some dare devils may be willing to risk life and limb, but you don't need to. Wear a helmet or appropriate headgear any time you are doing any activity where there is the possibility of falling and hitting your head like horseback riding, surfing, skiing, skating, or riding in all-terrain vehicles. Choose a sports program that enforces rules for safety and avoids drills and plays that increase the risk for head impact.

As far as possible, avoid exposure to radiation, toxins, poisons, any substances known to be harmful to brain or body, and transmissible infectious diseases. Avoid substances that may damage the brain's neuronal control centers.

Protect your mind. Avoid exposing it to negative pictures, images, or ideas that might return to disturb sleep, trigger nightmares, or any undesirable behavior that might result in injury—like falling out of bed or falling down the stairs.

Protect your lungs. Inhale fresh air, minimize exposure to pollutants such as tobacco smoke, vehicle exhaust, and fire smoke. Wear a mask if air quality is poor.

Protect your ears when around loud sounds. Protect your eyes when involved in activities that could trigger flying debris.

Avoid distracted walking and driving. Many get into accidents during distractions.

Protect your digestive system from low-quality foods and beverages—from *anything* that could diminish its effectiveness.

Wear a seat belt every time you are in any type of motor vehicle. Never drive while under the influence of alcohol or drugs.

Fall-proof your home. Remove throw rugs and other tripping hazards. Use a sturdy stepstool when reaching for high objects. Be careful with ladders—stay off them and off the roof. (Leave that to the experts!)

The first time you do something, your brain lays out the outline of new software in case you want to do it again. The good news is that this makes repeating that behavior easier. The bad news is that the brain can end up developing some bad habits because you "did something once."

A smart man only believes half of what he hears. A wise man knows which half ... Safety is something that happens between your ears, and not something you hold in your hands.

—Jeff Cooper

The NFL acknowledges that repetitive trauma to the head in football ... can cause a permanent, disabling injury to the brain. —Bob Fitzsimmons

An ounce of prevention is worth a pound of cure.

—Benjamin Franklin

Making safe, wise choices about brain-body safety means that you are planning for a healthier future. What you do today determines where you will be tomorrow.

*****

Healthy exposure to sunlight can boost the production of serotonin, the happy hormone that also makes you feel calmer and more focused and optimistic. The sun always shines above the clouds.

—Paul F. Davis

11 - Laughter as Medicine

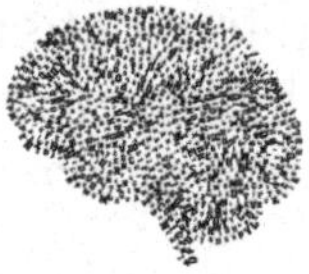

Mirthful laughter is a miracle medicine that requires no health care visits, special prescriptions, clothing, or environment.

Think of laughter as a form of play for both your brain and body—while also being very beneficial. An interesting phenomenon, laughter is considered a form of audible speech, arising from Broca's Area in the brain's left frontal lobe. Emotions, feelings, affirmation, and derision can all be conveyed through laughter.

Humor is a mental faculty located in the right cerebral hemisphere. If you have honed your sense of humor, it typically activates when something you did not expect to see, hear, or think occurs. Humor may be triggered by seeing someone skid on a banana peel or hearing a child or pet make unusual sounds or seeing a funny cartoon, or you name it. The identified humor can then trigger laughter

Choosing to laugh disengages regular life, which may not be very humorous at that moment. Laughing from your diaphragm helps rid the lungs of residual air, makes room for deep inhalations of fresh air, can be relaxing, and tends to be catching!

When sustained laughter comes from the inside, the brain *gets* it and releases endorphins, dopamine, and serotonin to help you feel better. Just a verbal recognition of "that's funny" does not seem to trigger the same release of brain feel-better chemicals.

Studies suggest that adults need a minimum of 30 mirthful laughs a day for good health. Very happy people tend to laugh 100-400 times a day. Very happy children tend to laugh 400-600 times a day—unless told to "Stop being silly!"

Laughter exercises are helpful for older adults. In one study, laughter improved the short-term memory of adults over the age of 65. Simply anticipating humor decreased their cortisol levels by nearly 50%.

Laughter can be *reflexive*. It is virtually impossible to control laughter when you are being tickled playfully—something you can't accomplish alone. (Try to tickle yourself and there's no surprises and no laughter!)

Laughter can also be *instinctual,* as in hearing the unexpected punchline on a joke. This appears linked with the hypothalamus. You may or may not be able to control instinctual laughter, especially if you're being told to "stop laughing." Good luck with that!

Female humor tends toward word play in the left hemisphere and stories about something that strikes their funny bone. Females connect through language, but rarely through jokes. Male humor is more right-brained. They use jokes and slapstick humor to connect with each other and with good friends. Males tend to tease people who they like.

Learning each other's humor *is* possible—and doubles one's triggers for laughter. Humor and laughter promote healthier relationships. Couples who laugh together tend to stay together.

Much like yawning, laughter is an intensely infectious activity that triggers the Brain Reward System. Dr. Madan Kataria of India found that when groups of individuals get together and *choose* to just start laughing, it soon turns into genuine laughter. Be serious about life but avoid taking every little thing too seriously. Develop your sense of humor! Stand in front of a mirror and practice laughing out loud.

Hang out with people who have a good sense of humor and love to laugh. You don't feel like laughing? Choose to laugh anyway and keep at it. A cheerful mind works healing. Laugh and *last*. If you are too busy to laugh—you are too busy!

Laughter brings increased oxygen to the brain and activates the release of anti-stress hormones that allow you to function more efficiently and joyfully. —Dr. Otálvaro

Laughter is the shortest distance between two people. —Victor Borge

Nothing can stand against the assault of laughter. —Samuel Clemens (Mark Twain)

Laughter is the most inexpensive and most effective wonder drug. Laughter is a universal medicine. —Bertrand Russell

He who laughs at himself, never runs out of things to laugh at. —Epictetus

As soap is to the body, so laughter is to the soul.
—Jewish Proverb

You don't stop laughing when you grow old, you grow old when you stop laughing.
—George Bernard Shaw

Humor is by far the most significant activity of the human brain. —Edward de Bono

*****

Encourage one another and build each other up. —The Apostle Paul

12 - Support Group

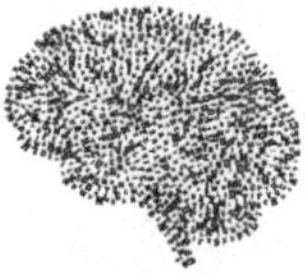

John Donne's statement that no one is an island ... each is a piece of the continent comes from his book "Devotions upon Emergent Occasions," published in 1624. It emphasizes the interconnectedness of humanity, suggesting that the loss of any individual may affect everyone.

Richelle E. Goodrich had a similar philosophy when she wrote that everyone needs a support group on which to rely—whether family, friends, therapists, or religious leaders. Human beings cannot live life alone and expect to stay mentally, emotionally, and spiritually healthy.

Each human being needs a few individuals who "have their back." Since you are the only person who will be with you for your entire life, your relationship with yourself is of paramount importance. Equally so, that small circle of trusted individuals with whom you feel free to share joys, hopes, puzzlements, sorrows, and genuine love.

Those with a good support system tend to be healthier and live longer than those who don't. In one survey, the average female identified nine people with whom she could easily relate.

The average male identified one or none. If one, he usually identified his spouse. No wonder studies have shown that divorce can be emotionally devastating for a male—he loses his one support person.

Greek Philosopher Epictetus believed that the key is to keep company only with those who uplift you, whose presence calls forth your best. Your close friends can enhance or sabotage your success. Align yourself with those who:

- Exhibit a healthy superego and practice meaningful and consistent self-care.
- Create and maintain a positive mindset and effective self-talk patterns.
- Have a good sense of humor and laugh easily and a lot.
- Are wise and supportive, making healthier choices with the future in mind.
- Study, learn, turn information into knowledge, and apply it daily.
- Embrace and live a healthy lifestyle.

Water seeks its own level and so do brains and behaviors. Identify the type of person you want to have around you and then develop some of those skills. As you mature, you will naturally be attracted by and become attractive to those who are on a similar life journey. These are the type of individuals you want for a support group.

According to Jim Rohn, you are the average of the four or five individuals with whom you spend the most time. Studies estimate that within three years you are at risk of adopting their habits, especially happiness, smoking, health, and obesity. They may adopt yours, as well. Unfortunately, negative habits appear easier to copy than healthier positive habits.

A support group is about relationships. However, giving and receiving is a tricky equation. Relationships in a support group need to be reciprocal—never a one-way street either in giving or receiving. Sometimes you give; at others you receive.

Individuals with an overinflated sense of self-worth are often comfortable taking but not giving. Those with an underinflated sense of self-worth often give endlessly but are uncomfortable receiving. That equation needs to be in balance. If you lean toward an extreme, work to develop balance.

When someone wants to give you something in friendship and you dismiss their efforts—you deprive them of the opportunity to feel good about what they were able to do and wanted to do for or with you. This could be viewed as a self-centered choice.

Do you feel unworthy? Do you feel over-entitled? Do you want to avoid owing anyone for anything? If so, you may have some family-of-origin work to do along with some growing up.

The value of relationships with those you love and who love you—your *support group*—is inestimable. Many have said that what they most regret in life is not what they *did* but what they didn't do, the friendship opportunities they failed to appreciate and nurture—until it was too late. Select the members of your support group with great care. Be intentional and wise about who, how, and when you choose to engage with others. Stay alert to keep your life in balance.

If you want to go fast, go alone. If you want to go far, go together. —Old African Proverb

True love is rare, and it's the only thing that gives life real meaning. —Nicholas Sparks

Friends are angels who lift our feet when our own wings have trouble remembering how to fly.
—Unknown

*****

I get great satisfaction from trying to get better and from trying to do the next thing as well as I can. —Brad Stevens

13 – Stressor Management

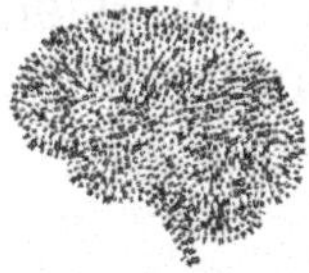

Dr. "Hans" Selye, a Hungarian Canadian endocrinologist, took the descriptive word *stress* from the field of engineering and applied it to human beings. Dr. Selye taught that in many cases it is not the stressor that kills human beings, it's their reaction to the stressor. Richard S. Lazarus, PhD, defined stress as a condition, sense, or feeling that is experienced by individuals who perceive that the demands upon them exceed the personal and social resources they can mobilize.

Stress can be triggered by internal or external factors. According to Dr. Al Seibert, no stress exists in any situation unless an individual human brain perceives something as a stressor and experiences strain. The resulting *stress* is less due to what occurs or exists objectively and far more due to the way in which the brain perceives what is happening.

Epictetus, a freed slave and 2nd century Greek philosopher, taught that it isn't so much what happens to you that matters but what you *think* about what happens. This is often referred to as a 20:80 Rule. Only 20% of any negative impact on your brain and body is due to the identified stressor. At least 80% is due to your perception of the stressor and how much weight or importance you choose to give it. While you may not be able to prevent the 20% in any given situation, you can do everything about the 80%, because your brain creates your perceptions.

Distress and misstress impact both perception and flexibility. Estimates are that fully 50% of all the stressors with which humans grapple are of their own making based on how they think. Many react to perceived stressors using beliefs and attitudes that were absorbed before the age of five or six years old. The adulthood goal is to embrace *Eustress* (positive stress that helps you grow) and minimize negative *Distress* and often hidden negative *Misstress.*

Once a stress response has been activated, estimates are that it takes about 72 hours for the body to return to a state of homeostasis or balance—if the individual has implemented effective stress-management strategies. The length of the stress response can be extended by ruminating on undesirable aspects of a situation or by disclosing and rehearsing your discontent to any who will listen.

Ask yourself: "How much will this event, situation, or stressor matter in twelve months?" If there is a high probability that it will matter, do the work to brainstorm and problem-solve. If it won't matter, let it go!

Studies have shown that fear and thankfulness cannot co-exist in the brain. *Gratitude* trumps fear. Think of something for which to be grateful, and that will be the focus of your memory.

Stress is as unique as your brain and your fingerprints. The hippocampus, the brain's search engine, is especially sensitive to stressors. Chronic stressors can shrink and even destroy brain cells in the hippocampus.

Your perception of the stressor and learned reactions, degree of flexibility, level of emotional intelligence, ability to be serious about life (while not taking every little thing *too* seriously), along with acquired "tools and strategies," all influence the stressor's impact on your life and the results you experience in your brain, body, and relationships over time.

Identify your triggers, perceptions, stress patterns, reactions, exhibited behaviors, and consequences. If your stressor strategies are resulting in negative outcomes, craft and implement healthier responses.

Chronic stressors tend to increase cortisol levels, that increase cravings for high-fat, high-sugar comfort foods, which trigger a cycle of emotional eating, that results in fat storage around the abdomen, which can lower testosterone levels and increase estrogen production in both males and females. None of these is a good thing.

Every good mood you experience is your decision, and so is every bad mood. Everything you do in anger is your decision, and so is everything you do with love and compassion.
—Ralph Marston

The greatest weapon against stress is our ability to choose one thought over another.
—William James

If you are distressed by anything external, the pain is not due to the thing itself, but to your estimate of it; and this you have the power to revoke at any moment. —Marcus Aurelius

One person's pleasure is another person's pain.
—Old Proverb

*****

Success is a measure as decided by others. Life satisfaction is a measure as decided by you. —Old Proverb

14 - Life Satisfaction

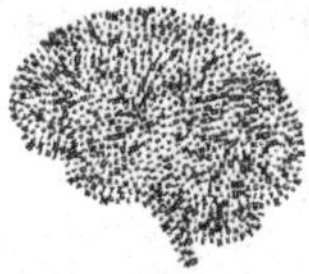

Life satisfaction is one of the most decisive factors for staying healthier and younger for longer. However, it is more complex than many realize. Although some suppose that life satisfaction is a synonym for happiness, it represents a separate concept. Life satisfaction involves the evaluation of one's life as a whole and not just a recognition of a current level of happiness or accomplishment.

Life satisfaction seems to come from within the brain based on personal values and what the individual believes is important. Multiple studies in various cultures have shown that an emphasis on materialism such as money, possessions, affluence, social class, things you own, technology, and even who you pride yourself on hanging out with, does not appear to be linked with higher levels of life satisfaction.

A balanced sense of self-esteem also plays a definite role in influencing life satisfaction. This includes understanding that you have value simply because you exist. Identifying ways in which you have contributed positively to the lives of others in your community reinforces an affirming mindset and self-talk style that is related to overall life satisfaction.

Both hope and optimism are linked with higher levels of life satisfaction, as does a mindset that looks favorably on one's life and overall accomplishments rather than depending on one's current, fleeting, or momentary feelings.

An "attitude of gratitude" has been linked with life satisfaction. Thankfulness has been shown to help an individual learn to delay immediate gratification, a critical requisite for almost any type of success. Those who wrote "gratitude letters" to others who had made a difference in their lives were found to score higher on scales of happiness and lower on scales of depression—and the effects lasted for weeks!

The emotion of Joy in the left hemisphere cannot simultaneously coexist alongside anger, fear, or sadness, the protective emotions in the right hemisphere. A mindset of joyful thankfulness promotes congruence of thoughts, emotions, and feelings, which tends to increase life satisfaction, reinforce gratefulness, improve problem solving, provide an antidote for fear, and enhance both health and potential lifespan.

Life satisfaction appears to increase with age, especially as individuals become wiser and more knowledgeable, and practically apply what they have learned. Interestingly, studies have shown that morning-oriented people ("larks") tend to show higher levels of life satisfaction than do evening-oriented people ("night owls").

Those with high levels of life satisfaction typically exhibit a positive mindset and a good superego. They tend to take good care of themselves and are also concerned with the well-being of others. They take appropriate steps to keep their own "cup" full. This allows them to share from an overflowing supply rather than from a deep well of unmet needs.

Characteristics of those with good life satisfaction include a balanced sense of self-esteem, an ongoing sense of hope, a decision to choose joy and contentment, and a high EQ that helps avoid or minimize conflict.

Hone your spirituality, the spirit with which you live life. Do something every day to evoke a sense of awe in your brain and heart; then pass it on. It only takes a moment to smile, to lift someone's spirit, to make a positive difference in another person's life and, in the process, make a positive difference in your own life.

Find ways to give back to Planet Earth, its inhabitants, and the environments needed to sustain life. Think ahead. Do whatever you can to help ensure a quality life for the next generation, and the next, and the next.

Disciplining yourself to do what you know is right and important, although difficult, is the high road to good self-esteem and personal satisfaction.

—Margaret Thatcher

Gratitude unlocks the fullness of life.

—Melody Beattie

Be thankful for what you have, and you'll tend to end up having more. —Oprah Winfrey

Satisfaction is knowing that you're doing the best that you can. —Lydia Lunch

Personal satisfaction is the most important ingredient of success. —Denis Waitley

Do right always. It will give you satisfaction in life. —Wovoka

80% of life's satisfaction comes from meaningful relationships. —Brian Tracy

*****

Chronic stress is now considered a risk factor for Alzheimer's disease. Cortisol floods the brain during stress. When the stress never stops, neither does the cortisol. PET Scans have revealed that the prefrontal cortex and the hippocampus are the first to suffer under relentless stress.

—Urja Vohra, 2025

15 - Alzheimer's & Prevention

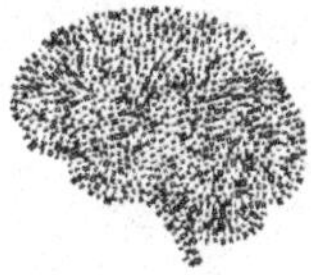

Alzheimer's disease (AD) was named for Dr. Alois Alzheimer, who noticed changes in the brain tissue of a woman who had died of an unusual mental illness that included memory loss, language problems, and unpredictable behaviors. More than a century later, no cure for Alzheimer's disease is in sight. Some scientists, however, have turned their research to identifying prevention strategies.

According to the National Institute on Aging, in most cases Alzheimer's appears to be a lifestyle disease. It can be influenced by genes in combination with epigenetics, which is everything that is not genetics. There are five main types of dementia.

- Vascular, involving high blood pressure.
- Alcoholic, related to alcohol use.
- Parkinson's, with Lewy bodies in brain cells.
- Frontotemporal dementia, brain shrinkage.
- Alzheimer's, 60-80% of current dementias.

Every 65 seconds, someone in the US is diagnosed with Alzheimer's. The Alzheimer's Association estimates that over seven million Americans aged 65 and above are living with Alzheimer's disease, which is the most common cause of dementia. Almost two-thirds are of those diagnosed are female. The cost is approaching $350 billion dollars annually. By 2050, estimates are that one in every three adults in the US may be experiencing dementia symptoms or will be caring for someone who is.

Studies have identified 10 common symptoms.

- Memory loss.
- Challenges in planning or solving problems.
- Difficulty completing familiar tasks.
- Confusion with time or place.
- New problems with spoken or written words.
- Misplacing things and can't retrace steps.
- Decreased or poor judgement.
- Withdrawal from work or social activities.
- Changes in mood and personality.
- Trouble understanding visual images and spatial relationships.

Two diagnostic strategies—a PET scan and a sampling of cerebrospinal fluid—now allow physicians to identify plaques and tangles with a reported 95% accuracy. A 2024-2025 review updated risk factors for dementias including Alzheimer's. Some are preventable, others must be identified and managed.

- Depression
- Diabetes
- Insulin resistance
- Lower education levels
- Obesity

- Smoking, vaping.
- Untreated vision loss
- Air pollution
- Alcohol use
- Family history of dementias
- High Blood pressure
- High LDL cholesterol
- Physical inactivity
- Social isolation
- Traumatic Brain Injury
- Untreated hearing loss
- Unmanaged chronic stressors
- Brain inflammation

Factors that trigger brain inflammation have been identified. They include the following.

Alcohol

Avoid alcoholic beverages, including red wine. Go for non-alcoholic beverages. In 2023 the World Health Organization stated: There is no safe amount of alcohol consumption that does not affect health."

Aluminum

Unquestionably neurotoxic, aluminum has been found in all Alzheimer's brains that have been studied. Prevent aluminum products from touching your food. Use stainless steel cookware or those that have a ceramic coating that is listed as being “free of PFAS, PFOS, PFOA," identified as "forever chemicals."

Chronic Stress

High stress levels negatively impact the brain’s glymphatic immune system and the body’s general immune system. Higher chronic stress levels pour cortisol into the brain and body. PET Scans have shown that this can create inflammation, which can damage the prefrontal cortex and the hippocampus—areas highly involved in memory functions. Scientists have noted that most young people these days are under constant stress related to education, financing, and job hunting. How this will impact a risk for dementia is of increasing concern.

Nutrition

Lean toward a DASH or Mediterranean eating style. Include nuts and legumes, whole fruits and vegetables prepared as naturally as possible, and sourdough bread made with natural starters. Minimize refined and processed foods due to the sugar, salt, and fat content. Avoid fried or barbequed foods (heat-altered fat increases inflammation). Avoid fast food and its wrapping paper as it may contain PFAS. Avoid red/processed meats (sulfites), saturated, hydrogenated, or trans fats.

Fructose

The brains of those in early Alzheimer's contained high levels of fructose. Avoid the use of any High Fructose Corn Syrup (HFCS) by any of its 15 or so names. It is 100% fructose.

The brain uses glucose to generate energy. Obtain it from healthier carbohydrates and foods that typically are lower on the Glycemic Index, such as avocado, almonds, walnuts, seeds, whole grains; whole fruits as only 1-2% of ingested fructose reaches the brain; vegetables such as broccoli and legumes,

Refined Sugar

Minimize the use of refined sugar as it is 50% fructose and is added to many prepared foods, especially "low fat" prepared shelf foods, to (reportedly) make them more edible. Avoid added refined sugar, high salt, and chemical additives.

Water

Estimates are that 75% of Americans are chronically dehydrated—especially those over age 60 as thirst sensations diminish with age. Just a 1% level of dehydration—and you are not yet recognizing any thirst—results in a 5% loss in cognitive ability. Make your beverage of choice the purest water you can find. In 2024, NIH issued conclusions following a major review of hydrogen water studies: "Hydrogen-Rich water (HRW) offers several potential strengths, including its antioxidant, anti-inflammatory, and anti-apoptotic (cell-death) properties."

According to Franziska Spritzler, RD, CDE, a growing body of research suggests brain insulin resistance is strongly linked to Alzheimer's. Learn to read labels. Carry a small magnifying glass, if necessary. Usually, the shorter the list of ingredients the better.

For most people, prevention strategies likely will require lifestyle changes. Choosing and maintaining preventive changes can be a challenge but it is doable. Compared with Alzheimer's, prevention is the way to go.

*****

Your genes are not your destiny—your lifestyle is. —William Li, MD

The term *research* means "to search again." Why not? Sometimes, a new interpretation emerges that is of utmost importance.

—Isaac Asimov

16 - Genetics & Epigenetics

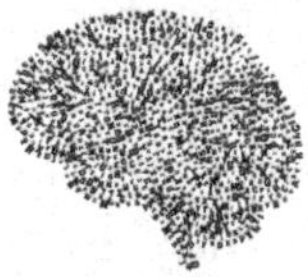

You arrived on Planet Earth with a genetic inheritance in place known as your *genome*. You didn't put in an order for your specific genome, but it's yours anyway—kindness of your two biological parents. Genetics is believe responsible for about 30% of your level of health, wellness, and your potential lifespan.

Your unique genome includes chromosomes and genes. A 1962 Nobel Prize was awarded for the discovery of the molecular structure of DNA, known as the double helix. Estimates are that 99% of your DNA is located in your chromosomes. The remaining 1% is found in the mitochondria, tiny energy factories inside cells that have a clearly defined nucleus. You inherit mitochondria from your biological mother only. The mitochondria create ATP (adenosine triphosphate), the energy source needed to power almost all cellular activity.

Some 25,000-30,000 genes (not 150,000 as once thought) are tiny bits of DNA that contain "genetic blueprints" for creating you. They determine your inherited traits such as body build, height, type of hair and its color, the color composition of your eyes, your skin tones, along with your potential talents—or brain *bent*—that you can develop and hone over your lifespan. Estimates are that during the first trimester of gestation, more than 95% of embryos form correctly, based on their genetic blueprints. The embryos that do not form correctly may born with a birth defect.

By the end of the first 12 weeks of pregnancy, the initial construction of body organs is in place. These include brain, heart, lungs, digestive system, liver, kidneys, and the circulatory system with its arteries, veins, and capillaries. It also includes the body's immune system and the brain's glymphatic immune system.

The brain continues to develop throughout pregnancy with neurons being created at the rate of 250,000 per minute. More than half of all fetal metabolic energy is devoted to growing the brain, which will continue to develop and mature for years after birth, some believe perhaps until late thirties or early forties.

Genetics is only part of the story. Epigenetics, one's epigenome, includes everything that is not genetics. It is believed to account for about 70% of a person's level of wellness and potential lifespan. Epigenetics starts impacting the fetus the moment the father's sperm unites with the mother's egg or ovum and will continue to do so over an individual's entire lifetime.

Vital nutrients, hormones, and chemicals are carried from the placenta to you, the fetus, via the umbilical cord. These substances provide you with information about what is happening to your mother physically and emotionally. In whatever way she experiences her internal and external environments—dreadful or delightful—your will share the impact of her experiences.

Uterine scans have identified at least four core emotions that can be seen on the face of the fetus during pregnancy that reflect what the mother is experiencing emotionally: joy, anger, fear, or sadness.

It is believed that the fetus is able to sense the mother's emotions and feelings. In all likelihood it may also sense whether it was a wanted pregnancy and if it is the male or female child that its parent(s) hoped for. Some researchers think that the fetus also is able to sense at some level if it is a failed abortion attempt.

If both biological parents were present and a united, supportive team, the mother's emotional wellbeing was more likely to be positive. If the parents were unhappy about the pregnancy or if for some reason the father died or was separated from the family, or abandoned the mother, her emotional wellbeing may be less likely to be positive.

The fetus may sense if the maternal and paternal family systems are excited about the pregnancy and are eager to welcome the newborn with open arms. If not, the fetus may sense potential danger in the external environment.

When a pregnant woman perceives something as stressful, the stress response is triggered automatically. This results in substances such as adrenalin and cortisol flooding her body. Her developing fetus receives that information, too. If the stress response is triggered frequently, the fetus can become hyper-sensitive to any type of event or situation that it perceives as stressful.

This pattern can continue after birth, resulting in a tendency to *overreact* in stressful situations. Once the stress response is triggered it can take up to 72 hours for the body to return to a state of balance or homeostasis. If the stress is chronic, maintaining a desirable balance can be seriously undermined if not impossible.

Studies with mice led by Tracy Bale, PhD, at the University of Maryland, School of Medicine, have shown that it is not just maternal stress that can impact the developing fetus. Negative and/or chronic stressors can alter the father's sperm, which then can potentially impact the development of the fetus.

Epigenetics may also help to explain the *rage* that some abandoned, foster, surrogate, or adopted children may exhibit. Their new environments may be very different from the environments they became accustomed to during pregnancy. Healthy or unhealthy it was familiar, including smells, tastes, sounds, touch, music, language, race, culture, or even location on the planet. A disconnection from what was familiar can be stressful and unsettling, for the newborn.

Each person develops a mindset that Carol S. Dweck, PhD, describes as usually either "fixed" (life is what it is and there is nothing you can do about it) or "growth" (you are able to impact your own life by your lifestyle choices). Your perceptions come from your mindset. They influence how you perceive and interpret life.

In your teens and on into adulthood, you can review your perceptions: analyze them, keep some, dump some, tweak some, and create new ones. You can alter your mindset and your perceptions negatively or positively, which impacts epigenetic signals that are transmitted to components inside your cells. These signals influence how genetic blueprints are read and interpreted, and how building blocks are fashioned and repaired.

Who you are as a unique individual involves complex interactions in your brain and spinal cord, your microbiome and virome (the bacteria and viruses—good and bad—that live inside you), and your genome and epigenome. It can also include behavioral cellular memories passed down from the past three or four generations of biological ancestors.

A common perception for generations was that a newborn's brain entered the world as a relatively blank slate. Current wisdom has turned that upside down. It is now believed that a newborn brain is far more developed, aware, and perceptive than anyone ever imagined!

This tiny brain can remember voices, songs, and stories it heard during gestation; understand a great deal of spoken language, communicate easily through sign language long before speech is produced; and learn two or three different languages simultaneously—as long as one parent speaks one language consistently, the other parent speaks a second language consistently, and another family member (e.g., a grandparent or frequent caregiver) speaks a third language consistently.

This relatively new body of knowledge about biology may help explain how specific diseases and behaviors occur more often in some family systems: cancer or heart disease, diabetes or strokes, lung problems or liver failure, addictive behavior tendencies, and even your risk for developing dementia.

It is also clarifying what you can and cannot change in this complex genetic-epigenetic equation sometimes referred to as *nature* and *nurture*. Turns out, human beings can change quite a bit depending on their lifestyle choices.

Epigenetics is powerful and includes what happens to you, the choices you make, the habits you develop, the behaviors you exhibit, the stressors you are exposed to and how you respond, your job or career, and your relationships, both personal and professional. It includes lifestyle.

The lifestyle you develop can positively or negatively interact with your epigenome. In adulthood, you make choices every day (little and large) that create your lifestyle—which has a much greater impact on health and longevity than was once thought possible.

You cannot change the past, but you can create a healthier future for yourself and for any biological offspring you may have.

- Learn whatever you can about your genetic inheritance, as strategies may be available to reduce your risk for some illnesses and diseases.
- Choose a growth mindset.
- Evaluate your mindset, self-talk, and perceptions, and adjust them as needed.
- Develop a healthy longevity lifestyle.
- Prevent what is preventable and handle more effectively what was not or could not be prevented.
- Choose wisely, making decisions based on informed evaluations.
- Stop talking about the old behavior you want to alter. Talk only about the new behavior that you are embracing as if it's a done deal.
- Maintain vigilance. Correct your course immediately if you notice you're using an old unhelpful behavior.
- Use willpower to help you create and sustain new behaviors.

According to Daniel M. Wegner, PhD, willpower has been often misunderstood. It was not designed to help you stop an undesirable behavior, especially one that gives your brain some type of reward. That is the reason some studies suggest that attempting to use willpower to stop addictive behavior is often unsuccessful over the long term.

Fortunately, willpower was designed to help you select, develop, and persevere in implementing and following a new healthier, and more functional behavior; one that results in positive outcomes.

In childhood you likely had to follow the lifestyle chosen by your parents or care providers. In adulthood, you get to choose your lifestyle—if not in every particular, in many areas of life.

Epigenetics is powerful. Sometimes it can even override genetics, helping you to stay healthier and younger for longer.

The past is never dead. It's not even past! You carry it within you. —William Faulkner

Bottom line?

Lifestyle Matters!

There is a cult of ignorance in the United States, and there has always been. The strain of anti-intellectualism has been a constant thread winding its way through our political and cultural life, nurtured by the false notion that democracy means that "my ignorance is just as good as your knowledge."

—Isaac Asimov, PhD
Professor of biochemistry at Boston University and prolific American writer

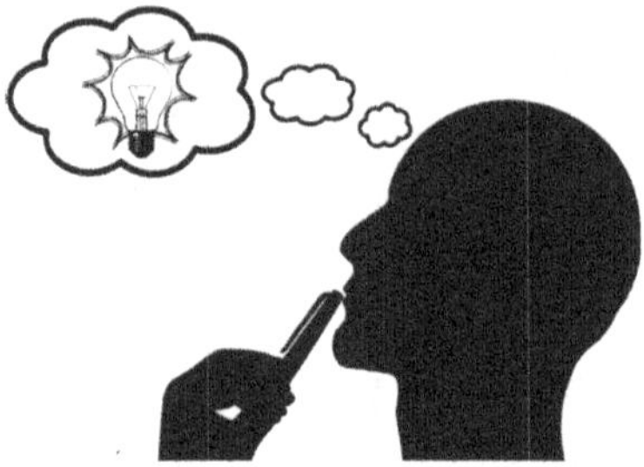

Keep questioning. Curiosity has its own reason for existing.

—Albert Einstein

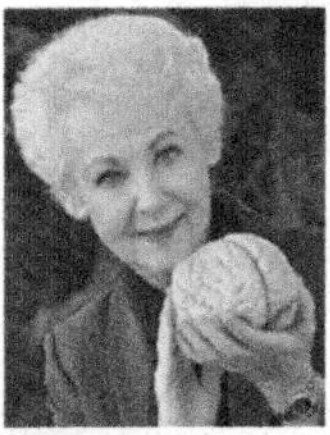

There has never been a brain on Planet Earth exactly like yours, nor will there ever be again. You are the only person who can live your giftedness—your brain's *Bent*—and if you fail to do so, the universe will be deprived of what only your brain can offer!

—Arlene R. Taylor, PhD

Brain-function specialist, author, musician, and internationally known speaker, Taylor is founder and president of Realizations Inc, a 501(c)(3) non nonprofit corporation that engages in brain-function research and provides related educational resources.

A sought-after presenter, Taylor is a recipient of the American Medal of Honor for Brain-Function Education from the American Biographical Institute Inc (#20/100, 2001). Taylor holds two earned doctorates; has life membership in the *National Registry of Who's Who*, 2000 edition; qualified for membership in Mensa International; and is a past member of the National Speakers Association.

Taylor's YouTube Channel:
www.youtube.com/@braingurutaylor/videos
Website: www.arlenetaylor.org
Contact: thebrain@arlenetaylor.org
Books are available at www.amazon.com

Each day I realize how much my own inner and outer life is built upon the labours of others, both living and dead, and how earnestly I must exert myself to give in return as much as I have received and am still receiving.

—Albert Einstein

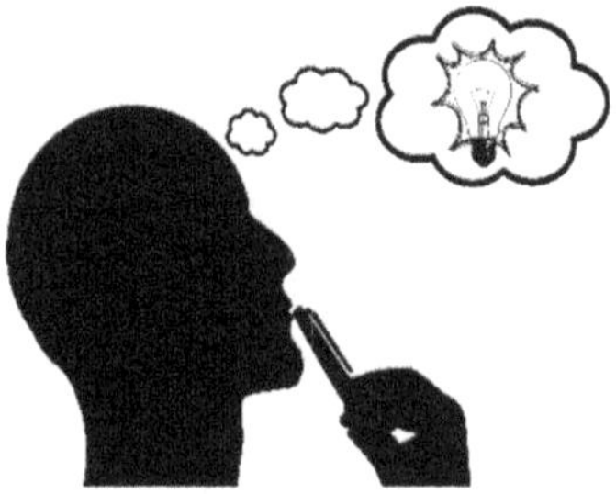

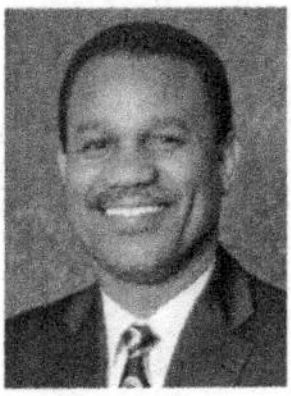

With appropriate motivation, education, practical application, and the right use of their brains, individuals may feel better, look better, think more clearly, and live healthier lives for longer.
—Steve Horton, M.Div., MPH

Horton is enthusiastic about health and wellness, believing that developing a healthier lifestyle matters. Not only is this possible, but it can also be effective and enjoyable. Even fun! His goal is to provide educational resources in a stimulating, easy-to understand, and practical-to-apply format.

As part of a lifelong commitment, the information and strategies can help people in the community become more aware of simple lifestyle changes to benefit their overall health, increase the likelihood of avoiding preventable diseases, and reduce symptoms of existing chronic illnesses.

Horton holds two earned master's. He promotes health and disease prevention locally and internationally.

Contact Horton at: stehor123@sbcglobal.net

If you don't sabotage the body's natural processes, your chances of making it to 120 are excellent.

—Walter M. Bortz, II, MD

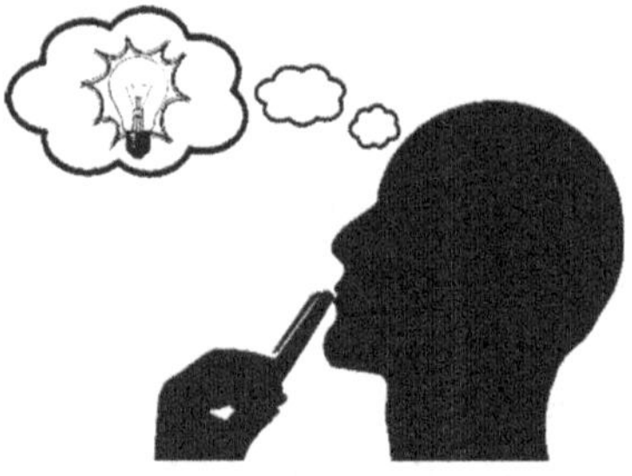

#1 - Case Study

The client, Mr. A.G., is an adult male with significant social and occupational responsibilities. His work involves extensive interpersonal engagement, writing, studying, and leadership. Prior to consultation, his lifestyle was marked by chronic stress and severe sleep deprivation. He had averaged two to four hours of sleep per night.

Mr. A.G. sought consultation after blood tests revealed prediabetes, with a reported HA1c of approximately 6.1. Although his glucose levels were not critically elevated, they were concerning. He also reported recurrent foot pain, particularly during periods of stress and lack of sleep. Additional contributing factors included minimal physical activity and dietary challenges, especially frequent exposure to inflammatory foods during social events.

Assessment identified chronic systemic inflammation as a primary driver of his symptoms, related to prolonged stress, inadequate sleep, limited exercise, and dietary patterns. The foot pain was considered an inflammatory manifestation rather than a direct metabolic complication. The primary intervention introduced was a daily lemon ginger drink, described as a low-dose, food-based anti-inflammatory beverage. Lifestyle education emphasized the inflammatory effects of stress, sleep deprivation, and inactivity, with encouragement toward gradual and sustainable changes, particularly improving sleep.

Within two weeks, Mr. A.G. reported resolution of foot pain. This improvement was sustained for nearly two years with consistent use of the drink. Missed intake was associated with symptom recurrence, reflecting ongoing inflammatory stressors rather than dependency.

Over time, Mr. A.G. increased sleep to approximately six hours nightly, resulting in improved mental clarity, reduced anxiety, a better focus on academic and clinical work, and deeper spiritual engagement. Reduced pain enhanced greater cognitive and spiritual functions, demonstrating the systemic impact of targeted lifestyle interventions. Longevity Lifestyle Principles applied included:

- Sleep optimization
- Inflammation reduction
- Stress management
- Habit consistency
- Mind–body–spirit integration

#2 - Case Study

The patient, Ms. L.R., is a 55-year-old female. She initially presented herself in a hospital setting after experiencing severe anxiety and physical distress following an allergic reaction to a prescribed medication.

Although laboratory tests and imaging were normal, she experienced intense panic and fear of dying. She was briefly admitted in error and discharged shortly thereafter.

During this encounter, elevated cholesterol and unhealthy lifestyle behaviors were identified, including vaping and alcohol use. She demonstrated high levels of anxiety, emotional distress, and panic.

Ms. L.R. was referred to a community-based lifestyle program. Initially skeptical, she followed up and attended regularly. The intervention emphasized gradual lifestyle modification, including rest, nutrition, physical activity, hydration, stress reduction, and spiritual practices. Group education, structured routines, and devotional activities incorporating prayer were central components.

Over subsequent weeks, Ms. L.R. demonstrated marked improvement. She discontinued harmful behaviors, including alcohol use and unhealthy social activities.

Follow-up with her physician showed normalization of cholesterol and other laboratory values. She reported weight loss, improved physical well-being, and a substantial reduction in anxiety and stress.

Mentally and emotionally, she became calmer, less irritable, and more emotionally regulated. She expanded her engagement beyond health classes to participation in worship services and structured spiritual study.

Because of limited prior exposure, foundational Bible stories were introduced to support understanding. Over time, her interest deepened, leading to participation in more comprehensive study. This case illustrates the interconnected effects of lifestyle change on physical, emotional, and spiritual health in an adolescent patient. Longevity Lifestyle Principles applied included:

- Lifestyle changes—first intervention
- Stress and anxiety reduction
- Community accountability
- Behavioral habit changes
- Spiritual resilience

#3 - Case Study

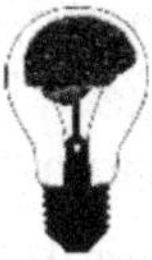

The client, Ms. A.K., is an adolescent female approximately 26-28 years old. She participated in a Longevity Lifestyle program alongside her mother. Prior to enrollment, she experienced symptoms consistent with prediabetes as well as significant depression and anxiety. Her symptoms included frequent emotional episodes, irritability, and reliance on social media rather than face-to-face relationships.

Ms. A.K. adopted lifestyle changes concurrently with her mother, following the same dietary patterns, physical activity routines, hydration practices, and rest principles.

The intervention emphasized a whole-food, plant-based diet, regular exercise, adequate water intake, stress reduction, and spiritual practices, including devotionals and prayer.

Over time, Ms. A.K. experienced substantial improvement in mental and emotional health. Episodes of depression and anxiety, which had previously occurred frequently and sometimes daily, became significantly less frequent. She became calmer, less irritable, and more emotionally regulated.

Her mother reported improved behavior and absence of prior anger and hostility. Symptom fluctuations were observed during lapses in adherence. Increased intake of sugar, animal products, and processed foods was associated with irritability and emotional instability.

When lifestyle principles were resumed consistently, her mental and physical stability returned.

Ms. A.K. developed healthier social behaviors, reduced excessive social media use, and formed meaningful in-person friendships. She reported improved happiness, greater engagement in church activities, and interest in using music and singing as a form of ministry.

This case highlights the bidirectional relationship between lifestyle behaviors and mental health. I demonstrated that sustained lifestyle interventions can support remission of both metabolic and psychological symptoms. Longevity Lifestyle Principles applied included:

- Nutrition for brain health
- Mental health through lifestyle changes
- Inflammation reduction
- Social connections enhanced
- Consistent adherence to protocols

#4 - Case Study

The patient, Mr. D.S., is a Hispanic male in his late 50s. He was encountered in a telemetry unit after admission for severe heart failure. He was diagnosed with cardiomyopathy of unknown cause, with a critically reduced ejection fraction of approximately 15%.

Mr. D.S. weighed nearly 300 pounds and experienced profound shortness of breath and functional limitation. Hospice care had been discussed due to poor prognosis.

Mr. D.S. and his family were in significant emotional distress. His mother was praying at his bedside, and his wife expressed fear and hopelessness. He was invited to participate in a lifestyle-based health program focused on heart recovery through comprehensive lifestyle modification.

Despite severe limitations, he attended consistently. Initially, he could barely walk short distances without stopping. Interventions were introduced gradually and included dietary change, progressive exercise, weight management, stress reduction, and spiritual practices. Dietary changes were challenging but sustained.

Over the following months, Mr. D.S. demonstrated dramatic improvement. He transitioned to regular exercise, eventually using a treadmill for up to an hour. He lost nearly 100 pounds within eight months. As his cardiovascular fitness improved, blood pressure and heart rate normalized, allowing reduction of heart failure medications under physician supervision.

Follow-up imaging showed recovery of cardiac function, with ejection fraction improving from 15% to approximately 55%, confirmed by echocardiography and cardiac MRI.

He returned to full-time work after a period of disability. Anxiety decreased, and he developed consistent spiritual practice.

This case demonstrates the potential for sustained lifestyle intervention to reverse advanced cardiac disease.

Longevity Lifestyle Principles applied included:

- Lifestyle medicine in severe disease
- Weight loss for cardiac recovery
- Progressive physical activity
- Medication reduction
- Mind–body–spirit healing

#5 - Case Study

The patient, Mr. H.T., is an older adult male estimated to be in his late 60s to early 70s. He was encountered as a hospital patient with a complex medical history, including a serious autoimmune-related kidney disorder with antibody-mediated damage to renal tissue. His condition had progressed to the point where plasmapheresis was required to remove circulating antibodies. He also experienced multiple complications, including pneumonia, and dialysis was being considered.

Mr. H.T.'s daughter believed he would benefit from lifestyle modification and encouraged him to attend a lifestyle-based health program. He agreed and began participating consistently. A structured lifestyle regimen was introduced, emphasizing whole-food, plant-based nutrition, gradual physical activity, hydration, rest, stress reduction, and spiritual engagement.

Over time, Mr. H.T. experienced substantial improvement. He lost a significant amount of weight and adhered closely to a plant-based diet. Follow-up laboratory testing showed marked improvement, leading to eventual normalization of kidney function. As his renal markers stabilized, plans for dialysis were discontinued. Steroid and immunosuppressive medications were also stopped as laboratory values remained within normal ranges. His blood pressure normalized as well. Challenges arose in coordination with healthcare providers, as some continued prescribing antihypertensive medications despite normalized blood pressure. Mr. H.T. eventually was able to reduce unneeded medications and reported feeling much better.

Functionally, he returned to activities he had previously abandoned due to illness. He resumed part-time work as a mechanic and returned to music, an important personal pursuit. He also became a regular church attendee, engaging socially and spiritually. Clinicians described his recovery as a "miracle," though it coincided with consistent lifestyle adherence. This case demonstrates the potential for lifestyle-based interventions to support remission and functional recovery in advanced autoimmune and renal disease. Longevity Lifestyle Principles applied included:

- Lifestyle intervention (chronic) disease
- Plant-based nutrition for renal recovery
- Weight loss for metabolic/kidney health
- Medication reduction via improved lifestyle
- Family support and advocacy
- Functional recovery and purpose restoration
- Mind–body–spirit integration

#6 - Case Study

The patient, Ms. L.M., is an adult female with a complex medical history, including type 2 diabetes, hypertension, mental health challenges (anxiety and depression), and a background of significant childhood trauma. When first encountered in a community health setting, she participated informally, primarily observing lifestyle coaching sessions and gradually implementing changes on her own.

Ms. L.M. adopted a structured lifestyle regimen that emphasized plant-based nutrition, regular physical activity, hydration, stress management, restorative sleep, and spiritual engagement. Over time, Ms. L.M. achieved substantial improvements in her health.

She lost significant weight, estimated at over 50 pounds, leading to normalization of her blood sugar and blood pressure. Her diabetes medications, including insulin and metformin, as well as antihypertensives, were progressively tapered under supervision and eventually discontinued. She also stopped medications for autoimmune or inflammatory disorders, such as steroids and immunosuppressive drugs, as her clinical indicators normalized.

Mentally and socially, Ms. L.M. experienced a profound transformation. She reported reduced anxiety and depression, improved interpersonal trust, and a newfound capacity for meaningful social connections. This, in turn, allowed her to re-engage actively in community and spiritual life. She began teaching, preaching, and serving in church activities, demonstrating increased confidence and functionality.

Her recovery illustrates the interdependence of physical, mental, and social health. Lifestyle interventions not only reversed chronic metabolic and cardiovascular conditions but also facilitated emotional healing, social engagement, and spiritual growth. Clinically, her case demonstrated a potential for non-pharmacological and holistic approaches to produce measurable and sustainable improvements in both body and mind, even in patients with complex, longstanding health challenges. Longevity Lifestyle Principles applied included:

- Plant-based nutrition for health
- Weight management for systemic recovery
- Medication reduction via lifestyle adherence
- Exercise, hydration, and restorative sleep
- Stress management, mental health support
- Social connection, purposeful engagement
- Spiritual development and service

#7 - Case Study

The patient, Ms. R.N., is an adult female estimated in her early 60s. She experienced a significant injury after slipping and falling at a restaurant, landing on her back. Although imaging did not reveal fractures, she developed severe and persistent back pain consistent with soft tissue trauma, muscle strain, and inflammation. The pain was intense and long-lasting, significantly limiting her function and quality of life. She believed her condition would not improve and at one point felt she might not survive due to the severity of pain.

Ms. R.N.'s condition placed her at risk for chronic pain and potential dependence on pain medication, a common outcome in similar cases. Instead, she was introduced to a structured lifestyle-based recovery program that focused on reducing systemic and localized inflammation. A key intervention was the use of regular hydrotherapy treatments, applied to improve circulation and decrease inflammation in the affected area. These treatments were administered consistently over time.

Ms. R.N. adopted dietary changes, transitioning to a whole-food, plant-based diet to reduce inflammatory contributors. She also engaged in gentle movement and walking as tolerated, gradually rebuilding strength and mobility. During this period, she was temporarily removed from smoking exposure while participating in the program, which further reduced inflammatory burden. Over time, Ms. R.N. experienced pain reduction and functional recovery. Her mobility improved so that she was able to resume physically demanding activities, including outdoor labor (e.g., gold prospecting), which required endurance, strength, and sustained movement. This marked a dramatic contrast from her earlier belief that she would not recover.

Her case illustrates how targeted lifestyle interventions—inflammation reduction through hydrotherapy, nutrition, movement, and removal of harmful exposures—can support recovery from chronic pain and trauma-related musculoskeletal injury, even when conventional imaging shows no acute structural damage. Longevity Lifestyle Principles applied included:

- Inflammation reduction, basis for healing
- Hydrotherapy to enhance circulation
- Plant-based nutrition for tissue repair
- Movement for musculoskeletal health
- Avoidance of smoking
- Non-pharmacologic pain management
- Functional restoration and resilience

—The End—

or

—The Beginning—

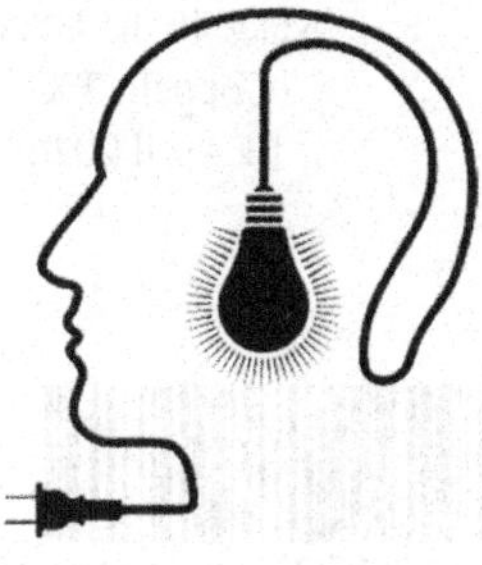

Made in the USA
Coppell, TX
14 April 2026

75543929R00056